Telehealth Security: An Examination of Variance in Telehealth Security Breaches

DR. SERIA D. LAKES

Printed in the United States of America

First Edition

ISBN-10: 0692291865
ISBN-13: 978-0692291863

Aires Designs
P.O. Box 473
Upper Marlboro, MD 20774

www.airesdesigns.com

DEDICATION

For Mom and Dad

CONTENTS

LIST OF FIGURES

PREFACE

Security in telehealth is often not given the adequate attention necessary to truly protect patient data. Telehealth provides major benefits such as faster and easier accessibility to medical records, health care consultations, and health care procedures. It is imperative for telehealth systems to be properly secured, since PII data is processed and stored on these systems.

This book examines the evolution of security implementations and policies for protecting telehealth data and provides details pertaining to telehealth in regard to: security, the technology of telehealth, potential frameworks, and HIPAA. Ensuring that communications occur securely is essential since telehealth is most notably dependent on wireless and electronic media to protect the quality of telehealth, data, patients, and practitioners.

There are several solutions that support the protection of telehealth data. Data encryption is the main protection factor that is stressed in current telehealth system protection solutions. National Institute of Standards and Technology (NIST) 800 series special publications provide guidance for implementing such security controls, especially in regard to encryption. However, encryption is noted only as addressable in HIPAA policies (U.S. Department of Health & Human Services, 2013a). Additionally, though HIPAA has *some* required security regulations, it is lacking in standards such as the implementation of a breach violation standard. The consequences of data breaches in telehealth can be as severe as financial or criminal penalties, legal ramifications, and identity theft. A breach standard, incorporating facets of encryption solutions as security requirements, might help serve as a more concrete guideline as to the security measures that telehealth facilities need to implement.

In addition, this book presents research that identifies prevalent breach types and mediums that are often involved in breaches. Telehealth breach rates between 2009 (when the

HIPAA Breach Notification rule was enforced) and 2012 were examined. Industry feedback pertaining to the implementation of policy reform in regard to thresholds was also gathered. Discovering the variance in telehealth breaches over this given time period, will allow for a better understanding as to how telehealth regulations can be improved, provide an understanding of typical breach amounts over a given period of time, and provide a foundation for suggesting a breach threshold in future research studies.

To conclude, this book provides a recommended breach mitigation process, as well as recommendations for possible HIPAA improvements. As technology evolves, there are opportunities for regulatory documentation to be improved. These improvements would potentially aid in providing better data security for evolving telehealth systems. The information presented in this book serves as a catalyst for more extensive research regarding the implementation of better telehealth security standards, threshold requirements, and governance.

ACKNOWLEDGEMENTS

First and foremost, I dedicate this book to my Lord and Savior, Jesus Christ. Without his grace this effort would not have been possible. I also, especially, dedicate this book to:

My loving parents, Elvoid Lakes III & Sherry K. Lakes – Thank you for bringing me up in such a way that I had the discipline to complete this endeavor. Thank you for encouraging me and keeping me motivated. I appreciate and love you more than words can express.

Ryan T. Taylor – Thank you for being my best friend and significant other. I love you and I appreciate your support, you being my cheerleader, and making me laugh when I need it most.

I also could not write a dedication without acknowledging the Lakes & Johnson/Connor families and, especially, my Grandparents Peggy L. Connor and Bobby J. Connor. Thank you for taking part in the responsibility of raising and shaping me. Denise, Whitney, Allison, Nancy, Dawn, Ejiro, Lauren, & Lareatha- "thank you for being a friend". My godson, Kaiden, I pray that you are happy and successful as you grow. Joy Lynn, thank you for being my perfect little companion. Finally, I dedicate this book to my Grandparents: Elvoid Lakes II, Jurlean Lakes, and James Henry Johnson; and my Uncle William Sullivan Jr. I appreciate the relationships God allowed me to have with you during your time here. I love you and hope that you are smiling down on this accomplishment.

There were several individuals who were instrumental in helping me to complete this milestone: Dr. Andrews – Thank you for being such a supportive and encouraging mentor. I know you spent a lot of time and effort in ensuring that I made it through my doctoral research. I greatly appreciate you. Thank you for all of the encouraging conversations that kept me motivated!

There are other professors in my past that I must

acknowledge, as well: Mrs. Dibler, Mr. Renwick, Mr. Savoy, and Mr. Young. Though years have passed since I graduated from High Point High School, your influence still has a profound effect on me.

Thank you all. God bless.

INTRODUCTION

Sitting in the doctor's office waiting area, I see a little girl around the age of 7 or 8 sitting in a chair swinging her legs. Her feet are too short to touch the ground. She persistently asks her mother if she can get a lollipop out of the basket at the front desk. This doctor's office is very tech savvy and makes use of electronic tablets to record patient data. New patients complete forms with the tablets, as well. All of the vitals go into the tablets. Patients are impressed with this seemingly simple solution to filling out numerous forms. Names go in, addresses go in...social security numbers go in. Unfortunately, as we're sitting in the waiting area, this sweet little girl, unbeknownst to us, is being attacked. Cybercriminals have hacked into the facility's portal and gained her social security number. The worst part about this situation is the fact that she, or her parents, may not even realize the impact of this attack until she goes to apply for a college loan a decade from now. There is often a sense, that "it will never happen to me", but it can...and it does happen to the "invincible" every day. As we continue to

evolve electronic health systems, these attacks will become more

prevalent. This battle will definitely leave scars that the doctor

won't be able to fix.

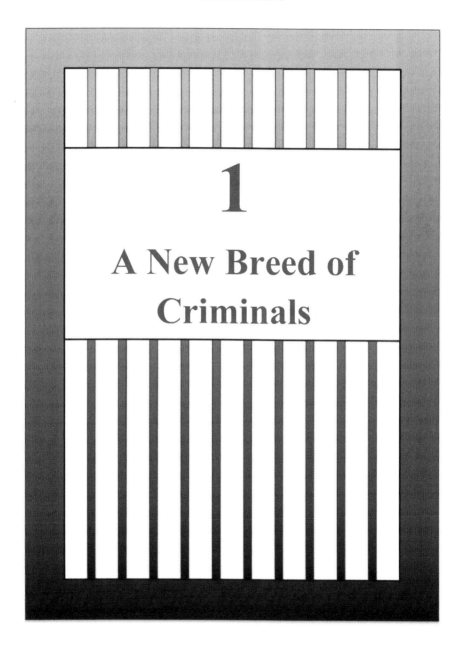

1

A New Breed of Criminals

CHAPTER 1: A NEW BREED OF CRIMINALS

Cybercrime is an important facet behind why the security of data transmitted in health information technology (HIT) exchanges is so crucial. Since telehealth involves the transfer and storage of personally identifiable information (PII) or data transmitted during procedures, such as telesurgery, ensuring the security of telehealth infrastructures using Internet protocols and establishing a standard as to what an acceptable breach amount should be, is even more pertinent than the security and standards required for general Internet use.

Telehealth is defined as the processing of patient information over a network to remotely provide patients with treatment, preventative health care, and consultation. This growing field relies on data transmission to deliver remote health care and its communications rely on procedures that outline the wireless and electronic handling of data. Over the past decade, advances in technology have influenced how data in health care and medical procedures is transmitted, communicated, and conducted. As telehealth grows, security breaches will become more prevalent. The establishment of an acceptable amount of security breaches may serve as an asset in motivating facilities to ensure adequate security measures.

Telehealth has existed in varying forms, over the past several decades, such as in the early uses of telephone and radio communications for health care consultations. The exact start date of telecommunication utilization in health care is unknown; however, more advanced uses of telecommunications began with the first remote surgery performed in 2001. The introduction of remote surgical operations to perform wireless health care and consultations in Transatlantic areas enabled modernized health care services to be received in areas where health care facilities were not present. Using this alternative method to deliver health care services enables areas that lack health care facilities or medical expertise to receive the benefits of modern health services.

Though the terms telemedicine and telehealth are often

used interchangeably, there is a distinction between the two functions. Telemedicine refers to the remote delivery of clinical medical services, using IT and electronic systems (American Telemedicine Association, 2006). Whereas telehealth refers to the remote delivery of clinical and non-clinical services which can extend to any technological attribute in support of remote healthcare, such as distance learning and outreach programs (American Telemedicine Association, 2006). Often both telemedicine and telehealth incorporate uses of similar technology, such as portals and distance monitoring tools (American Telemedicine Association, 2006).

Figure 1. Telehealth vs. Telemedicine

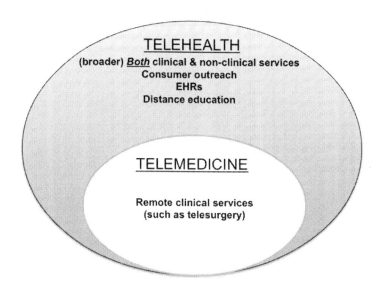

The vast majority of healthcare facilities, 94%, have suffered a security data breach since 2010 (Charette, 2012). Health Information Portability and Accountability Act (HIPAA) defines a breach as "the acquisition, access, use, or disclosure of protected health information in a manner which compromises the security or privacy of the protected health information" ("Breach Notification for Unsecured Protected Health Information", 2009, p. 42743). Protection of patient information and secure data transmission is important to the future of telehealth as it relates to patient confidentiality, as well as its ability to address the requirements outlined in the Health Insurance Portability and Accountability Act (HIPAA).

Telehealth spans the limits of medical phone consultations to telesurgery, and ensuring that HIPAA standards adequately provide accountability and secure coverage for all telehealth components is vital. Health practices are faced with the challenges of protecting patient data. HIPAA standards instituted by the Department of Health and Human Services (HHS) have been set in place to help ensure that patient data is securely transmitted. Insufficient policies that do not address the various facets of this type of health care can be costly, detrimental to patient health and health records, and could prompt legal ramifications.

The history of telehealth spans from past uses of telegraphs and telephones to the National Aeronautics and Space Administration's (NASA) efforts in further developing telehealth to medically aid astronauts in space travel. The increased usage of information technology in medicine has contributed to an increase in the overall amount of data breaches in medicine. The issue brief, "Privacy and security in healthcare: A fresh look (Issue Brief)" (2011), stated that the lack of regulatory policies and the lack of enforcement of policies are two of the reasons for the increase in breaches. The three major problems that organizations may face when involved with data breaches are financial penalties, flawed reputation, and loss of business. It is also noted that a third of data breaches in medical data transmission result in identity theft (Deloitte, 2011).

A major issue in telehealth is that insufficient security controls are often used. Additionally, there is an issue in the fact that there is a limited number of individuals with the necessary technical expertise to address cyberterrorism and security issues. This leaves telehealth systems vulnerable to attacks from computer worms and viruses. Telehealth, as a whole, is not given enough focus.

Licensing and legal issues, potential issues of patient privacy, lack of support from insurance entities, and lack of expertise in this new approach to administering health care are also issues. Though there are benefits, such as reduced cost and greater accessibility to health care, the somewhat impersonal interactions in telehealth could have the potential to negatively impact physician-patient relationships. Telehealth could improve efficiency and decrease health care costs; however, a level of trust amongst patients and providers must be established in order for telehealth to be widely adopted.

Research studies on the state of Telehealth security

Based on the lack of resource material pertaining to securing telehealth infrastructures, security is not a primary focus in regard to telehealth. If telehealth security aspects do not receive further attention, it will be difficult for people to adopt telehealth. A lack of attention on important security issues will impact the quality of telehealth care.

Regulatory tolerances have been established in other

industries, such as with U.S. government thresholds for procurement costs and poverty. The HHS makes use of the Consumer Price Index for All Urban Consumers (CPI-U) on an adjusted yearly basis to set the poverty threshold for the United States (U.S. Department of Health & Human Services, 2011). Likewise, the U.S. Department of Housing and Urban Development has developed statistical criteria to establish the Day/Night Noise Level (DNL) threshold for noise coming from roads and train tracks (Environmental Criteria and Standards, 2007). Just as these standards have established numerical thresholds, a telehealth breach acceptability standard would aid in motivating facilities to appropriately secure data in efforts to not exceed telehealth breach tolerance levels.

The Health Information Technology for Economic and Clinical Health (HITECH) Act and the American Recovery and Reinvestment Act (ARRA) add further safety controls to enrich HIPAA's policies. ARRA, often referred to as the "stimulus package", was introduced to stimulate the economy. It provided financial incentives to stimulate the economy in regard to education, infrastructure, energy, federal taxes, unemployment and welfare programs, and healthcare. In efforts to promote the move to developing technology-based healthcare systems and fair distribution of the health care funding provided under ARRA, the HITECH act was born.

The HITECH Act was passed as a component of ARRA in 2009 under the leadership of President Barack Obama. Technology has since evolved and HITECH seeks to protect technology infrastructures used in telehealth that were previously not covered under HIPAA. HIPAA was passed in 1996 under President Bill Clinton. Currently, telehealth facilities are required to abide by sanctions outlined in both HIPAA, HITECH, and in some cases, FISMA policies. There are several grant programs that resulted from HITECH, and one of the primary incentives under the HITECH act is that it gives states the ability to gain some of the ARRA-allotted money for healthcare in the form of grants, once it is identified that a state has adopted and implemented a telehealth infrastructure. States are required to develop strategic and operational plans in support of this, as well.

Additionally, federal agency implementers of telehealth infrastructures must abide by the Federal Information Security Management Act of 2002 (FISMA). FISMA requires federal agencies to develop & implement IT security plans to protect their respective IT systems. NIST developed Federal Information Processing Standards (FIPS) to support FISMA. FIPS requires federal agencies to report IT security results, annually, to the Office of Management & Budget. Since telehealth employs the use of IT systems, adherence to FISMA is necessary, for federal agencies implementing telehealth infrastructures.

Figure 2. HIPAA, HITECH, ARRA Relationships

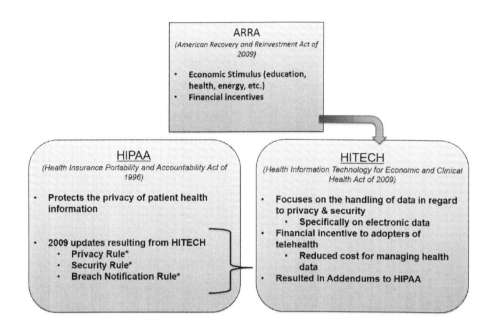

Background of the Problem

    Telehealth has revolutionized how health care is administered and the possibilities for rural telehealth could be endless in regard to the accessibility of health care. Funding to support telehealth infrastructures has become more prevalent as the benefits of telehealth are demonstrated. Approximately $20 million has been spent by the U.S. Department of Veteran Affairs on the installation of telehealth monitors in over 16,000 homes in the United States (Nagy, 2006). The Defense Advanced Research Projects Agency (DARPA) funded a $12 million initiative to develop Trauma Pods, or pod structures with remote surgical components, to deliver remote surgery to U.S. military personnel.

While trauma pods and telesurgery may be financially unattainable for many rural areas; a good, cost efficient start to implementing telehealth infrastructure into the home of rural residents would be video conferencing . Since many households currently possess a computer, applications that can be used with existing household computers, tablets, or mobile phones can be leveraged. The establishment of telehealth capabilities via mobile applications and at public locations has been beneficial in providing greater accessibility to health care resources. As a result of telehealth, medical expertise is now readily accessible to areas that previously did not have close access to healthcare. The protection of such telehealth capabilities, especially in regard to breach acceptability standards, is essential to the continuance of telehealth.

While there are several benefits that telehealth provides to society, the cost and effectiveness of security implementations and cybercrime are problematic factors regarding telehealth. Internet protocols are used for data transmission during telehealth communications. Since Internet protocols, such as hypertext transfer protocol secure (https), secure sockets layer (ssl), and secure shell (ssh), are used for telehealth data communications (see NISTIR 7497 Guidance on Encryption); security risks are a concern that must be considered.

Questions for Discussion and Exploration

1. Identify and discuss 3 telehealth cybercrime incidents in the last year. How could they have possibly been prevented?

2. Identify a U.S. state's telehealth strategic or operational plan. Identify how it could be improved.

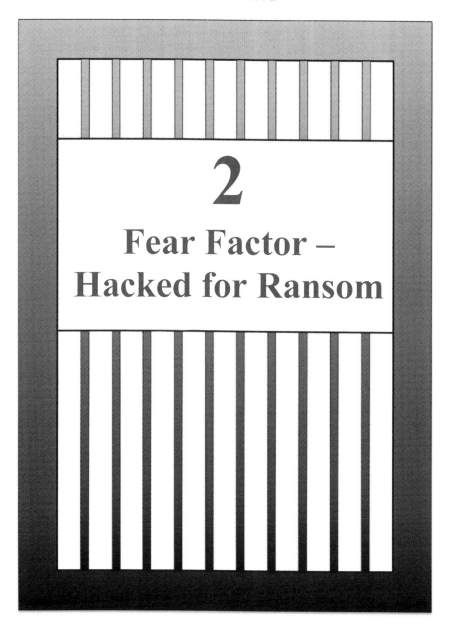

2
Fear Factor –
Hacked for Ransom

CHAPTER 2: FEAR FACTOR – HACKED FOR RANSOM!

A 2014 survey conducted by the Ponemon Institute (2014) revealed that 90% of the organizations that were surveyed reported a telehealth breach in the last 2 years and 38% reported more than 5 breaches in the same time period. This is a mild decrease from the Ponemon Institute's 2012 study in which 94% of organizations reported a breach and 45% reported more than 5 breaches (Ponemon Institute, 2014). However, these numbers are still high. The fear factor associated with HIT breaches is that criminals are selling obtained information to other parties in underground markets. Once PII is obtained, criminals can perform malicious activities, such as: making fraudulent charges for services, ordering prescriptions for resale, opening financial accounts, accessing existing financial accounts, and blackmailing.

Cybercriminals are stealing telehealth data in expectation of the receipt of a ransom. Facilities practicing telehealth, such as Chicago's Surgeons of Lake County and Virginia's

Prescription Monitoring Program were both hacked for ransom in recent years. The amount requested for ransom in the Virginia's Prescription Monitoring Program scenario was an astounding $10 million. No ransom was ever paid in either of these scenarios; however, the damage of PII being accessed and obtained was already done. Scenarios such as these express the gravity of data security in telehealth transmissions, as well as the importance of effective telehealth documentation, such as operational plans.

If a telehealth system is not properly protected, network attacks and unauthorized disclosure could occur. An adversary could observe any data that the telehealth system sends out if a telesurgical device is attacked. An adversary could also observe any data that the surgical robot system receives. If this happens while a telesurgical operation is in progress, the system could be hijacked and remotely controlled by malicious parties. Possibly classifying certain telehealth related systems, as life safety systems may assist in elevating the importance of a higher need for strong security, especially in regard to encryption.

Denial of service attacks or man-in-the-middle attacks could be detrimental to areas of telehealth, such as telesurgery. Telesurgery is surgery that occurs remotely. Once an adversary gains control of a surgical robot and is erroneously cutting a patient, they can rupture arteries, stab the patient, and ultimately, kill the patient. It is inevitable that security breaches may occur, however, preventative security measures and breach acceptability standards need to be implemented in efforts to protect telehealth systems from such transmission attacks.

> # Why is this important?
>
> There is a good chance that you have medical data stored on your physician's computer/portal. The system could get hacked and someone could steal your identity...
>
> *This is important because it more than likely affects* *you.*

Though HIPAA and other health information exchange

(HIE) guidance documentation provide telehealth security requirements, these documents do not provide a requirement pertaining to an acceptable telehealth breach amount. Guidance for implementing security controls for the protection of telehealth data is provided in documentation such as NIST Special Publication 800-66 Revision 1 (see NIST Special Publication 800-66 Revision 1 Guidance for HIPAA required access control and transmission security) and NIST Special Publication 800-53 Revision 3 (see NIST Special Publication 800-53 Revision 3 Guidance on Access Enforcement); however, no acceptable breach amount is mentioned. Additionally, there are HIPAA standards regarding the privacy of patient information in healthcare; however, there is a concern by practitioners, patients, and governing entities; regarding the lack of HIPAA required regulations pertaining to telehealth standards for securing data. Though, HIPAA's Administrative Simplification Statute and Rules provides provisions regarding the lack of protections for privacy and lack of security controls for telehealth personally identifiable information (PII), a standard pertaining to an acceptable amount of security breach violations regarding these facets needs to be developed and enforced.

The REAL Problem

The general problem is that there are inadequate dedicated security controls to protect against network attacks, interference and potentially loss of life. The lack of security requirements in telehealth impacts the quality of care administered to patients. The specific problem is that the telehealth industry has not identified a tolerance level for the amount of breaches that will be considered as acceptable over a given period of time. This means that there is no "magic" number of enforcement that will result in an indefinite system decommission, after multiple data breach and/or hacking incidents.

Between 2009 and 2012, only 48 of the 50 states in the U.S. reported telehealth security breaches to the HHS (U.S.

Department of Health & Human Services, 2013a). Telehealth security breaches from any of these 48 states which reported a violation, as states are required to do, are included in HHS documentation (U.S. Department of Health & Human Services, 2013a). Reported breach records are posted on the HHS government website in the Breach Notification database. These records are considered public domain, and public access to this data is supported by the Freedom of Information Act (FOIA) and HHS regulations (Freedom of Information Act, 2009; Freedom of Information Regulations, 2003). The Privacy Act prohibits patient data from being recorded in this database (Privacy Act, 2013). An analysis of the Department of Health and Human Services (HHS) breach records could aid in identifying areas that need improved security requirements, as well as identify any variance that can provide an understanding of typical breach amounts over a given period of time. Inadequate security in telehealth could diminish the numerous benefits that this field is providing.

Telehealth provides several innovative benefits to society and will help to benefit both the Medical and information technology (IT) fields. This form of health care provides greater medical accessibility to patients and providers, as well as a faster communication means to aid in treatment. Telehealth has an influence on the advancement of secure IT communication and devices. Developers are further enhancing existing security mechanisms, which promote safer data transmission in regard to both telehealth and IT communications. Encryption is a significant security control that aids in protecting the confidentiality (see NISTIR 7497 Guidance on Encryption) of telehealth data.

HIPAA addresses several security facets, but only notes encryption as addressable or required only after a risk assessment deems it necessary (U.S. Department of Health & Human Services, 2013). For example, the HIE Challenge Program mentions security, but not specifically encryption. Likewise, the HIPAA Security Rule requires the implementation of encryption only after a risk assessment (see HIPAA Security Rule, 45 C.F.R. § 164.312) deems encryption as necessary for protecting telehealth PII ("HIPAA Security Rule", 2007). Though encryption is viewed as a significant security control to protect confidentiality of data, adequate encryption may not be implemented by some facilities because of the upfront implementation costs. Due to the importance of data confidentiality in telehealth, encryption is a security facet that should be required for all telehealth electronic transmission and storage.

It is essential to investigate potential information assurance threats and how they could negatively impact telehealth. The cost of being counteractive can be exponentially greater than the cost of appropriately and proactively implementing security measures. These counteractive costs could result in financial losses and loss of life. An initial enforcement of HIPAA's Breach Notification Rule is outlined in the document "How the Office for Civil Rights (OCR)

Enforces HIPAA Privacy & Security Rules"; however, a more extensive investigation into issues with telehealth security policies and the associated costs resulting from a lack of or flawed security controls is warranted. By examining telehealth security breach rates, it may be validated that an increase in telehealth security breaches typically occurs with each semi-annual time interval per calendar year. A typical increase may provide support for the argument that adequate encryption security controls need to be implemented, despite the upfront implementation costs. Moreover, a typical increase may support the need for an acceptable breach threshold standard and repercussions to be established and enforced.

Questions for Discussion and Exploration

1. Discuss whether encryption for telehealth should be required or whether it should remain as addressable.

2. List and explain at least 3 major issues that can result from a hacked telesurgery.

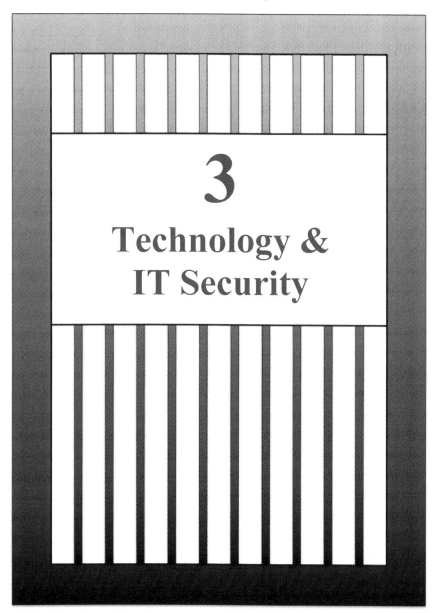

3
Technology & IT Security

CHAPTER 3: TECHNOLOGY & IT SECURITY

There are several factors that could diffuse the growth of telehealth and also stress the limitations of telehealth. The cost of communication links, data transfer rates, integration of technologies, organizational changes, and bandwidth issues are among many of the factors that can be viewed as limitations in regard to telehealth. Telehealth has prompted potential health care industry changes, to include: more demands for urgent care by patients, difficulty in assessments in diagnosis because of remote consultations, and health care fragmentation. The increased use of telehealth will prompt cultural, commercial, and operational changes. Various perspectives, such as management and economic perspectives; clarification of legal aspects; and government involvement are key factors that could negatively impact telehealth.

The trend of mobile communications is being increasingly used in the health care industry, specifically in regard to telehealth. 3G cellular technologies are providing avenues for telemedical communications that could not have been used in the past. 3G technologies allow greater telemedical communication, since they possess the capability of simultaneous and quick use of voice, data, multimedia exchange, messaging and computing.

A platform that supports telehealth communications and integrates advanced security for communications would be beneficial to the telehealth community. Cisco's application, called HealthPresence, incorporates these features. HealthPresence permits doctors to communicate remotely with patients via audio, chat collaboration, and video. The platform also allows doctors to monitor medical devices remotely. The HealthPresence platform has the capability to maintain up to 120 instances of the application on a single physical server to support multiple organizations, simultaneously.

HealthPresence boasts several security features that could be beneficial to telehealth facilities. The HealthPresence platform includes a failover mechanism, so that if a running server fails for some reason, all active processes will continue running seamlessly on a backup server. Security authentication can be performed by the platform using one of two methods: through the use of the platform's embedded technology or via Lightweight Directory Access Protocol (LDAP). Tools, such as electronic stethoscopes and otoscopes, will enable a doctor to assess a person's health at a distance. Physicians can perform many of the preventative health care techniques that would be performed in an in-office visit, just as effectively, using Cisco's telehealth platform, as well.

Though lower, pre-existing, quality-of-service connections can be used; often higher quality-of-service connections provide an overall better quality experience, as well as better reliability in regard to visual discrepancy, delay, and control latency. There are limitations related to compliance and legal ramifications; however, there are not yet concrete resolutions. Using network configuration and encryption to address the security and compliance of HIPAA is beneficial, and as barriers are overcome, the field will advance further and more widely (Hanley & Broderick, 2005).

Communication intrusion in medical devices communicating over wireless systems is also a potential issue in telehealth. NISTIR 7497 provides guidance on protecting telehealth architectures with the use of encryption (see NISTIR 7497 Guidance on Encryption); however, continuing to formulate and evolve protection mechanisms to negate such attacks in the future is imperative.

Electronic Medical Records (EMRs)

Several security experts are concerned with EMR platforms and applications, since health records are stored in one central location that is connected to the Internet. There are serious data security issues that could occur. While security experts have reason to be concerned about stored record security, there are far greater issues such as telehealth transmission incidents in hospitals that could result in patient death. A major problem lies in the lack of standardization in how organizations approach ensuring the security of data to satisfy security encryption guidance and policies. Due to the lack of standardization of security implementations, it is difficult to build and maintain relationships of trust between entities that need to exchange information.

Despite the security risks, the use of EMRs will allow greater access to health care, as well as decrease health care costs by $500 billion dollars over 15 years (Costa, 2007). EMRs also facilitate collaborative medical efforts among multiple physicians that work in different capacities, on an issue with a patient. Costa (2007) noted that while several other countries have moved to using EMRs, only about 20% of United States citizens' records are in an electronic format (Costa, 2007). Physicians and insurance companies already hold an individual's medical records, and data could be spilled or lost even in non-electronic formats by these entities.

Telesurgery

Two of the main devices used in telerobotic surgery are

the Zeus robot and the da Vinci robot. Telesurgery procedure types have evolved from open surgery, to minimally invasive, to robotic, and finally, to telesurgical. The team and elements required for telerobotic surgery include patients, surgical robots, robotic surgeons, telecommunication network and equipment, funding, and network engineers.

The da Vinci Surgical System Type S surgical robot is one of the tools that has revolutionized the area of telehealth. Utilizing telesurgical robots (TSRs), such as the daVinci, allows for greater accessibility to health care, reduced medicinal costs, and reduced time for procedural recovery. Da Vinci surgery can be seen in medical specialties, such as Neurosurgery, Orthopedics, and Urology. DARPA and NASA were the original financiers of the da Vinci surgical robot, developed by SRI International.

The da Vinci Surgical System Type S surgical robot was introduced to the public in May 1998 during the first robotic heart bypass surgery, performed by Dr. Friedrich-Wilhelm

Mohr at The Ohio State University. The first remote surgery was performed by the Zeus surgical robot and was performed in 2001 by Dr. Jacques Marescaux and Dr. Michel Gagner, who operated a console in New York, while the patient was in France.

Because of the limited resources to generate power for portable surgical systems in areas where health care is not readily accessible, such as war zones and areas where natural disasters have occurred, and ensuring that there are no issues with latency, jitter, packet delay, order, losses, and device failures; proper security controls supported by standards are essential to fluid operation. Due to the fact that surgical telerobotics systems operate wirelessly, they are more susceptible to network attacks from malicious adversaries. For example, security failures could occur if an attacker attacks the TSR and is aware that a smart card is being used, and attacks the smart card, as well. An attacker could take over a system and kill opponent soldiers, which is a prime reason as to why security in the operation of surgical telerobotics systems is so important.

Moving Forward

The engagement, privacy, security, and ability to financially sustain such an infrastructure are the most prevalent barriers. State-level efforts, such as the State Alliance for e-health, have been created to address the issues of interoperability; however, there is great importance in creating policies at the national level, so that cooperation in regard to HIT exchange can occur more seamlessly between facilities in different states. Cooper and Collman (2005) mentioned that a Kaiser Permanente facility in Northern California had 50% lower rates of death by heart attacks, than other facilities in the same region, due to Kaiser Permanente's use of data mining (Cooper & Collman, 2005). This has been attributed to the facility being able to provide patients with better care because its physicians can easily access a patient's complete health record during administration of health care.

Both the U.S. Department of Health and Human Services, as well as the Health Information Technology Standards Panel (HITSP) deemed the Certification Commission for Healthcare Information Technology (CCHIT) an accrediting body for telehealth. CCHIT's goal is to certify HIT products based on their security and interoperability aspects. Additionally, there are concerns with how HIPAA fails to address Regional Health Information Organizations (RHIOs). The results of a study by the Agency for Healthcare Research and Quality (AHRQ) emphasizes the inconsistent coverage and "patchwork" of policies and encryption guidance pertaining to HIT security and interoperability, as well (Desai et al., 2009).

Though the U.S. Government provides financial assistance for legislation, implementations of HIT can be costly. This may be a factor as to why there are not more HIT instantiations in facilities throughout the United States. Moreover, if HIT is used in addressing common chronic diseases, a foundation could be set to attract more individuals to adopt HIT as a means for improving the quality of health care.

Several encryption and security-based solutions are being

researched and developed. Some of these possible security

solutions use images, smart cards, RSA tokens, SSR-UDP;

Secure ITP/Interoperable Telesurgery Protocol (ITP), and

RFID. There are also hybrid solutions that are under

development.

Questions for Discussion and Exploration

1. Explain the pros and cons of the following solutions being developed: images, smart cards, RSA tokens, SSR-UDP Secure ITP, and RFID.

2. List and discuss 3 suggestions from NIST standards that can help protect telehealth systems.

3. Research and discuss DARPA and other government telehealth initiatives to help save individuals in war zones.

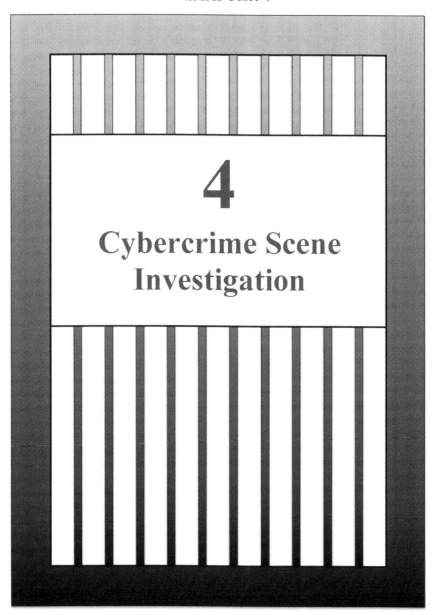

4
Cybercrime Scene Investigation

CHAPTER 4: CYBERCRIME SCENE INVESTIGATION

This book presents research that seeks to identify whether an increase in telehealth breaches typically occurred during each semi-annual time interval between 2009 and 2012. A typical increase in breaches per semi-annual time interval supports the argument that an acceptable breach level standard may be effective in requiring providers to implement proper security to reduce future breach amounts. HIPAA breaches reported to the HHS were broken into two major categories for this study: electronic mediums and breach type. The quantitative method used in this research study numerically displayed the breach levels regarding specific components; such as permissions, hacking, network, and email; in each of the reported HHS breach categories. Based on the analysis, this study provides a suggested telehealth breach mitigation process that could prompt providers to implement optimal security measures to better protect telehealth data.

Figure 3. Phased Study Approach

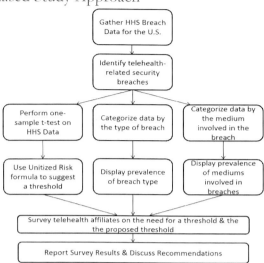

The study is grounded in the application of HIPAA

requirements for reporting breaches and the lack of a breach

acceptability standard. HIPAA regulations require telehealth

facilities to report breaches affecting 500 or more individuals to

the HHS, but there is not a threshold for breaches ("Breach

Notification for Unsecured Protected Health Information",

2009). A mandated acceptable breach amount regarding

telehealth should be an essential part of HIPAA requirements.

HIPAA policies should provide insight and mention the security

components that a state has or will implement regarding HIT or

Telehealth (Office of the National Coordinator for Health

Information Technology, 2009). An established breach standard would aid in ensuring the protection of patient PII data.

The facets of telehealth span communication from telephone consultations to distance remote surgery. To ensure data transmissions are protected, it is essential to ensure that security is adequate. Although HIPAA requires the implementation of security measures for telehealth facilities, the question as to whether or not these measures are adequate is relevant, because there have been a number of security incidents in this field just over the past few years (U.S. Department of Health & Human Services, 2013).

More than 50% of security breaches that occurred in the Mid-Atlantic states, between 2009 and 2010, were IT related (U.S. Department of Health & Human Services, 2013). Many of the breaches reported to the HHS were related to breaches of stored data (U.S. Department of Health & Human Services, 2013). This data is important because it shows a trend that medical facilities are not ensuring the security of their IT infrastructures, especially in regard to stored data.

Security for telehealth is often not given enough focus because of the additional costs that the implementing organizations would incur as a result; though the consequential costs of not ensuring proper security would greatly outweigh the costs of an initial proper security implementation. Moreover, the concept of using Electronic Medical Records (EMRs), though very beneficial in a multitude of ways, is also a security issue in regard to telehealth. The spillage of Personally Identifiable Information (PII) can be detrimental to both patients, as well as the facilities responsible for protecting the spilled patient data.

The geographic location of the study participants spanned the United States, and included any state that had a facility report a security breach. Not all states have reported breaches. The reporting facilities are in the District of Columbia and the following states: Alabama, Arkansas, Alaska,

Arizona, California, Colorado, Connecticut, Delaware, Florida, Georgia, Hawaii, Iowa, Idaho, Illinois, Indiana, Kansas, Kentucky, Louisiana, Massachusetts, Maryland, Michigan, Minnesota, Missouri, Mississippi, Montana, North Carolina, North Dakota, Nebraska, New Hampshire, New Jersey, New Mexico, Nevada, New York, Ohio, Oklahoma, Oregon, Pennsylvania, Rhode Island, South Carolina, Tennessee, Texas, Utah, Vermont, Virginia, Washington, Wisconsin, West Virginia, and Wyoming. Examining data that spans the entire United States was beneficial to this study, because it provided a thorough assessment as to how breach occurrences have varied since the instantiation of HIPAA's Breach Notification Rule in 2009. To identify prevalent characteristics of breaches, the study grouped data into categories pertaining to breach types and mediums. This data provided support for suggesting telehealth security improvements.

Experimental Procedures

Records from the Department of Health and Human

Services were used to identify the total amount of breach rates

per semi-annual increment. It must be noted that there are

limitations when analyzing HHS data with the goal of policy

improvement, namely due to: (a) a limited number of facilities

actually implementing telehealth, (b) the data reported to the

HHS only included breaches affecting 500 or more individuals,

and (c) the data that was assessed was limited to the categories

of breach types and medium types. The study was limited to

security breaches affecting 500 or more individuals, provided by

the HHS, due to the difficulty associated with gathering

accurate and timely data from multiple facilities in all states.

Using data from the HHS provided thorough and factual

information for the study. However, since HHS data only

included breaches affecting 500 or more individuals, results may

have varied for breaches affecting less than 500 individuals.

There were 595 records at the time of data retrieval from

the HHS website. Of the original 595 records, 438 records

pertained to telehealth in the 50 states in the U.S. and the

District of Columbia. There were 16 records pertaining to Puerto Rico that were removed, as the study focused on the continental United States. In addition, the following categories were removed, because they did not pertain to electronic media that connects to a network in transmission: Other (Backup Disks), Other (Backup Tapes), Other (CDs), Other (Hard Drives), Other (x-ray films), Paper, Paper (Mailing), and Paper & Films. There were 397 records, or 66.7%, that remained pertaining to the 50 states and the District of Columbia and were considered as using Information Technology, electronic format, or electronic media. These 397 records were the main premise for the research.

The HHS categorized data by the type of breach and the location of breach. The location of breach is referred to as the medium of breach for the purposes of this study. The categories for types of breaches were: hacking/IT incident, improper disposal, loss, other/unknown, theft, and unauthorized access/disclosure. The categories for breach mediums were: portable electronic device, laptop/computer,

network, server, other, electronic medical record (EMR), and

email.

Figure 4. Telehealth Breach Types & Medium Types

HHS Telehealth Data Breach Types	HHS Telehealth Medium Types
• Hacking/IT incident • Improper disposal • Loss • Theft • Unauthorized Access/Disclosure • Unknown	• Computer/Laptop • EMRs • Email • Network Server • Portable Electronic Devices

Several of the breaches spanned more than one category;

therefore, a category plot was used to total the amount of

breaches that pertained to each category. An analysis of breach

trends revealed an overall increase in breaches over the four-

year period that was examined. Figure 5 graphically displays these results.

Figure 5. Telehealth breach variance between 2009-2012

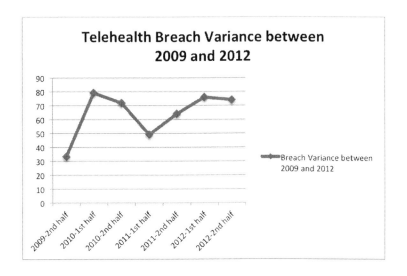

The research results show that, the hypothesis, *the total telehealth breaches for U.S. states will, on average, increase at least 20% of the time, based on semi-annual time increments*, is supported.

Laptop and computer related incidents, as well as network server incidents and portable electronic device incidents were most prevalently involved in telehealth breaches. The medium types of email, EMRs, and other stayed within a consistent range of less than 10 breaches per semi-annual

increment, over the period examined in this study. Additionally,

an increase was seen in portable electronic device breaches

toward the end of 2012. Incidents involving laptops or

computers showed the biggest fluctuation among all categories

over the four-year period. The breach count at the end of 2012

was near its highest breach rate since the instantiation of the

Breach Notification Rule.

Figure 6. Mediums involved in telehealth breaches from 2009-
2012

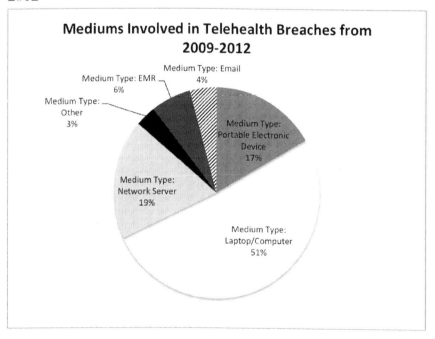

Figure 7. Prevalence of telehealth breach types from 2009-2012

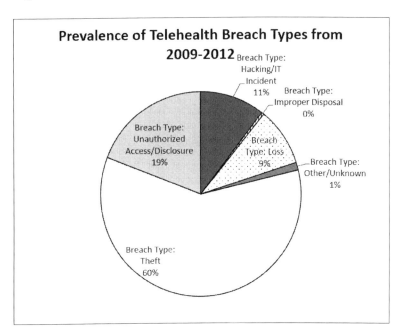

The frequency of breach types must also be noted. The categories of unauthorized access/disclosure, hacking/IT incident, loss, and other/unknown all remained within a consistent range of less than 20 breaches per semi-annual time period as displayed in Figure 9. There were only two documented telehealth breaches categorized as improper disposal. Therefore, improper disposal telehealth incidents only accounted for approximately zero percent of breaches.

The category of theft incidents was the most notable type of telehealth breach, comprising 60% of all telehealth breaches between 2009 and 2012, as displayed in Figure 7. This is a significant concern since the second most prevalent type of breach category was unauthorized access/disclosure, which accounted for only 19% of breaches as compared to the 60% of theft breaches.

Figure 8. Frequency of telehealth medium types from 2009-2012

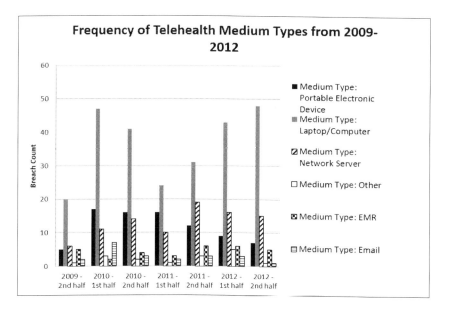

Figure 9. Frequency of telehealth breach types from 2009-2012

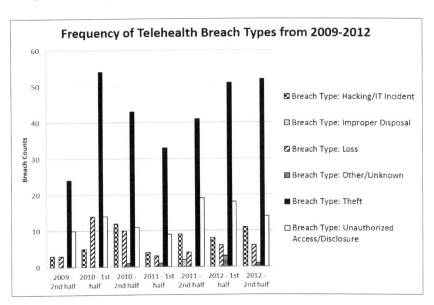

Medium Type

The study results revealed that in regard to medium

types involved in security breaches: 51% were related to a

laptop or computer, 17% of the security breaches were related

to portable electronic devices, 19% were related to a network

server incident, 3% of the medium types were documented as

other, 6% were due to the spillage of electronic medical records,

and 4% were related to email breaches. Several of the breaches

involved more than one type of medium. The results indicate

that more attention needs to be focused on the protection of data, especially in regard to the utilization of laptops and computer devices, portable electronic devices, and network servers.

The results show relatively maintained breach levels, over the longitudinal period, among most categories. However, the extreme fluctuation in laptop/computer breaches had a major impact in prompting the acceptance of the hypothesis.

The creation and enforcement of a security standard, specifically for telehealth communications, may influence breach rates where such a difference is negligible.

> **Did you know?**
>
> Breaches at the end of the study's research period were at one of the highest rates since the HIPAA Breach Notification Rule was instantiated.

Breach Type

Breach type analysis results appeared to have trends similar to those found in the medium type analysis results. The most prevalent type of breach, theft, decreased significantly from its initial peak breach count, in the first half of 2010, only to have increased to approximately the same peak level toward the end of 2012. This indicates the need for serious attention to be placed on creating and improving theft prevention security requirements.

The study results revealed that in regard to the prevalence of breach types among U.S. states: 60% of breaches were due to theft, 11% of breaches were a result of hacking or an IT incident, 19% were attributed to unauthorized access or disclosure, 9% were due to loss, and 1% were unknown. Improper disposal was an almost negligible factor in regard to any of the breaches reported to the HHS that dealt directly with telehealth. Both the most prevalent breach type of theft, as well as the category of unauthorized access or disclosure, indicates the need for better security mechanisms in storing data. The prevalence of hacking/IT incidents clearly shows that the existing security requirements, such as encryption discussions, included in HIPAA and in other telehealth advisory documents, are not adequately aiding in reducing breach levels. The results show that a more cohesive security infrastructure and structured standards for security telehealth facilities are necessary.

> **Security Issues!!**
>
> Greater security improvements are needed, especially, in regard to:
>
> *-Securing laptop & computer mediums*
>
> *-Preventing data theft*

It is clear that significant improvements need to be made in securing laptop and computer mediums, as shown in Figure 6.

Additionally, the study revealed that there is a significant issue with the high prevalence of data theft and that better requirements for proper security to prevent these forms of incidents need to be implemented, as supported by Figure 7. This study's data analysis results allows for a clear display as to areas where HIPAA needs to improve policies for protection.

Questions for Discussion and Exploration

1. Research the telemedicine/telehealth black market and identify reasons for why hacking and IT incidents are the most common types of breaches.

2. Identify 2 EMR platforms. Discuss the differences and similarities in the 2 platforms' security components.

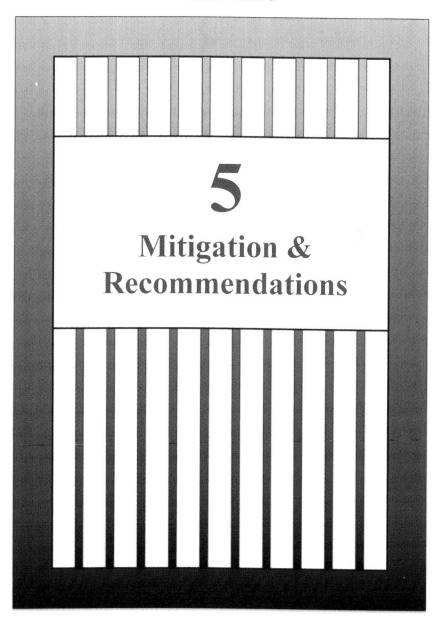

5
Mitigation &
Recommendations

CHAPTER 5: MITIGATION & RECOMMENDATIONS

The opportunities to improve HIPAA requirements could provide more secure telehealth systems and potentially decrease security breach levels. As telehealth expands it is inevitable that security standards may become more stringent. Improving the requirements of security in mandated policies and documentation could also help to reduce the number of telehealth security related breaches. The study presented in this book contributes to the body of knowledge pertaining to literature on telehealth security and breach thresholds, and should serve as a catalyst for expanding the knowledge base of how the adherence to adequate telehealth security documentation and standards may affect the prevalence of security breaches in telehealth.

Recommended Breach Mitigation Process

Based on research presented in this book, a hypothetical breach mitigation process has been designed that can be enacted once a HHS configuration control board deems the severity of breach significant enough to prompt some form of remediation. Once this proposed process is enacted, a facility has 90 days to submit a plan of action detailing how they will correct the issues based on NIST standards for security controls. The HHS will implement a configuration control board to review the plan and accept it or note where improvements need to be made for the plan to be accepted. If the facility does not comply with submitting a plan of action, there is a severe risk of the facility's telehealth systems being required to shut down. This decision will be made at the discretion of the HHS configuration control board. Once a plan of action is accepted, the involved facility will have 1 year from the acceptance date to have issues mitigated and resolved. If the facility does not comply with correcting the issues based on their plan of action, there is a severe risk of the facility's telehealth systems being required to shut down. This decision will be made at the discretion of the HHS review board, as well.

Although, logically, a decrease in breaches should

decrease risk, this may not always be true dependent on the severity of a breach. This process is presented to prompt policy development and discussion throughout the HIPAA security practitioner community. Threshold development based on breach severity, as well as security control requirements, are areas that could prompt future research studies. The recommended process is displayed in Figure 10.

Figure 10. Recommended breach mitigation process

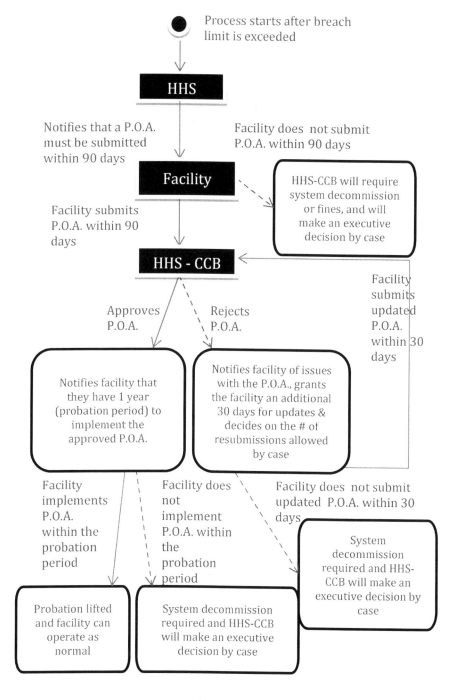

Industry Feedback

This study also considered the opinions of telehealth affiliates throughout the continental United States. Gathering the opinions of telehealth affiliates aided in gaining an understanding as to what, if any, breach threshold standards are currently being utilized among telehealth facilities. Telehealth affiliates were asked questions pertaining to their program or practice's use of methods used to quantify breaches, and whether external industry threshold benchmarks are being used.

There were 67 telehealth practitioners and affiliates that provided their opinions on the development of a telehealth breach threshold to aid in the protection of PII. Based on survey data, the prevalence of media used occurs in the following order: Laptop/Computer, Email, Electronic Medical Records, Network Server, Portable Electronic Device, and other. This may note the need for standards of various importance levels to be instituted based on the prevalence of each media category.

The feedback provided by telehealth respondents did not note any official threshold standards that were being used. When questioned about threshold standards used, some respondents noted that HIPAA and HITECH were used in their facilities to secure data. While these policies are relevant in regards to securing data, they do not include legislated breach thresholds. The recommendation of a threshold using another industry's may be a consideration for a future research standard.

Definitive responses from the market analysis were used to identify the level of support for such a threshold. The majority of telehealth associates, or 86%, were in favor of a legislated breach threshold for telehealth. Approximately 5% noted that they

> **Industry Feedback on Threshold Establishment**
>
> - 86% were in favor
>
> - 5% were neither for nor against
>
> - 9% were not in support

were neither for nor against the establishment of a threshold.

Lastly, 9% were not in support of a legislated threshold. A

response provided for lack of support noted that a threshold

could be cost prohibitive. The opinions of individuals

associated with the telehealth field were important in validating

the need for a threshold to be established.

Recommended Security Improvements

HIPAA policies consider several security mechanisms as

addressable, or in other words, required only after an initial

assessment shows the need. The requirements of these

assessments need to be clearly defined and included in HIPAA

policies to reduce vagueness. The first recommendation is that

encryption should be required for all telehealth systems, and not

just noted as "addressable". Though HIPAA requires

encryption to be implemented once a risk analysis presents the

need for such protection, encryption is not specifically stated as

being required for all systems transmitting data. Due to the fact

that some facilities in a state will require encryption, based on results of a risk assessment, a more detailed discussion on

encryption should be added to HIPAA.

In addition, a deeper correlation needs to be made in

regard to HHS documented breaches and possible

improvements for HIPAA. This valuable data should be used

to provide relevant and timely updates to security policies for

telehealth. Periodic reviews and analysis of breaches should be

completed. Based on the results from this analysis,

periodic security addendums should be added to constantly

improve HIPAA policies on telehealth security.

Breach-reporting data also needs to be more

detailed. The use of the documented categories as "other" used

for both the breach type and breach medium of a record should

not be allowed. A definitive category should be selected for at

least one of the breach characteristics. A thorough analysis

cannot be performed on data in which "other" is listed for both

the breach type and breach medium of a record. The addition

of the specific security mechanisms exploited and the type of telehealth occurring at each breached facility should also be documented. This will enable analysis to be performed on both the effectiveness of security mechanisms, as well as the types of security mechanisms needed to best protect certain types of telehealth procedures.

Data theft is a major root cause of telehealth data breaches followed by unauthorized access. Theft prevention can start with organization-enforced physical protection measures. Securing workstations, using strong cryptic passwords for data systems, and securing portable electronic devices in locked storage areas are seemingly simple, yet effective measures in physical protection. Shredding hard copies of access information and other sensitive should be enforced, as well.

In efforts to further safeguard the United States' sensitive data after the highly publicized breaches in 2013, the National Security Agency (NSA) implemented a two-man access control policy, also referred to as the "two-man rule", in which two authorized members of an organization are responsible for logging and monitoring when a portable electronic device is removed or returned from a storage facility. This has been implemented as an effective mitigation strategy in protecting classified data. Likewise, a two-man access control policy would be an effective measure in efforts to protect PII data from theft and loss.

There are also several commercial solutions that organizations can implement which consolidate multiple security facets into a single, easy to implement tool, such as an Intrusion Prevention System (IPS) and Unified Threat Management System (UTM). Intrusion Prevention Systems, combine the security features of detecting malicious intrusion on a network, as well as taking measures to prevent and negate further malicious activity. Data signatures, protocols, and typical network activity are all monitored to identify system abnormalities. Unified Threat Management Systems are advanced firewall systems that also include the capabilities of a virtual private network (VPN), data filtering tools, anti-virus applications, and data exposure prevention mechanisms. These consolidated tools would help aid in the prevention of both unauthorized access and hacking incidents

The final recommendation is that HIPAA needs to have a breach threshold standard. While penalty fines and criminal punishments are in place to encourage facilities to ensure the proper security of data, a threshold that may result in a facility's systems being decommissioned is an even greater motivator for a facility to truly ensure that patient data is secure. This study used statistical results to provide support for the development of a solution for this issue.

Questions for Discussion and Exploration

1. List and explain how a breach threshold could positively impact a reduction in telehealth breaches.

2. Explain why you think an explicit breach threshold has not yet been clearly outlined as a regulation.

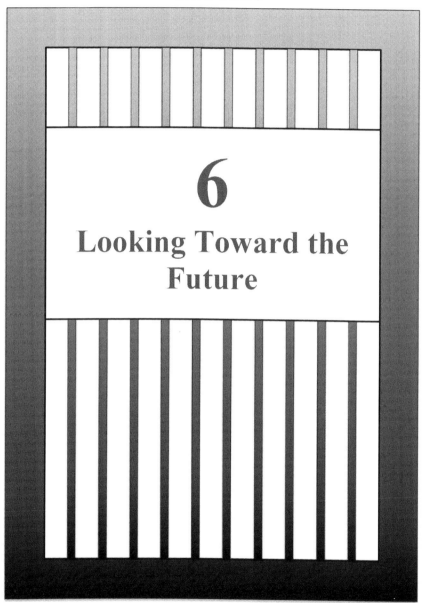

6

Looking Toward the Future

CHAPTER 6: LOOKING TOWARD THE FUTURE

Research supports the specific problem that the telehealth industry has not identified a tolerance level for the amount of breaches that should be considered as acceptable over a given period of time. While a tolerance level may not have yet been established, there are several mechanisms to protect data that could be integrated into HIPAA and other telehealth security documentation, such as HIE program operational plans. Additionally, this book revealed the detrimental effects of unauthorized access to PII, as well as its legal consequences. These factors stress the importance of documentation that requires proper security for telehealth systems.

Future recommendations specific to the effectiveness of existing telehealth security mechanisms include identifying the potential correlations between implemented security mechanisms and breach rates. An evaluation of the possible correlations that may exist between security mechanisms utilized and breach rate prevalence may prove valuable in identifying the necessary, optimal security controls needed to protect similar styles of telehealth systems. Similar styles of telehealth systems could be categorized into groups. The optimal controls identified for each categorized group of telehealth systems could then be, periodically, added to HIPAA as required security addendums. This would help satisfy efforts to provide adequate and timely security for each respective telehealth system group. A quantitative correlational research study may be the best research method to identify the potential relationship between implemented security mechanisms and breach rates.

Recommendations for future research, specific to mandated security documentation, include examining the possible relationship between telehealth security documentation and the breach levels of small telehealth facilities. Smaller facilities, which would include small medical practices, may experience breaches, but the breaches may have affected less than 500 individuals. Breaches affecting less than 500

individuals are not required, by the HIPAA Security Rule, to be

reported to the Department of Health and Human Services for

input into the Breach Notification repository. Gathering

information for breaches affecting less than 500 individuals may

be beneficial in identifying whether a relationship exists between

the adequacies of security requirements documented in HIPAA

policies and security breach levels of smaller telehealth practices.

A correlation may be identified that indicates that current

documentation positively influences breach levels for smaller

telehealth instantiations that maintain the data for fewer than

500 individuals. This could also prompt additional HIPAA

requirements for facilities based on the amount of patients

whose data would be used in a facility's telehealth

communications. Last, research that assesses the potential

correlation between security documentation and breach levels

by the amount of potentially impacted patients a facility has,

would add to the body of literature regarding the correlation and effectiveness of HIPAA documentation based on the size of a telehealth practice.

Conclusion

Telehealth is revolutionizing the way healthcare is administered and as result protecting data properly is essential to the continuance of this field (Coble et al., 2010). The results of the longitudinal research study in this book used statistical testing to reveal the acceptance of the hypothesis: that the total telehealth breaches for U.S. states will, on average, increase at least 20% of the time, based on semi-annual time increments. The goal of the study was to identify variance in telehealth breaches and provide support for the establishment of a breach threshold, since it would be advantageous in improving HIPAA policies. The study identified statistical difference among breaches, defined a proposed breach mitigation process, and identified industry support for the establishment of a threshold. Additionally, this study contributes to literature on telehealth security and the establishment of a breach threshold.

This study serves as a motivator for more extensive research regarding the implementation of better security standards and governance for telehealth. Future research includes examining how effective existing security mechanisms are in securing telehealth systems. Additionally, future research that examines the effectiveness of HIPAA in reducing the prevalence of breaches affecting less than 500 individuals may prove to be beneficial in identifying areas of necessary HIPAA improvements.

The advancement of distance healthcare, or telehealth, requires proper security to protect data and patient PII. Communications in telehealth are dependent on data being transmitted wirelessly and electronically. Although, states are legally obligated to follow policies set forth by HIPAA regarding security, telehealth is often implemented with inadequate security controls. Telehealth systems need to be implemented with proper security controls, so that systems are not left vulnerable to interference, cyber attacks, or unauthorized persons accessing patient data.

In response to the need to reduce data breaches in telehealth, as well as to properly protect patient PII data, HIPAA policies were developed (U.S. Department of Health & Human Services, 2013a). To further enhance HIPAA, a breach threshold should be developed and enforced. While telehealth presents great and convenient access to medical care for a population that may have had limited or no access to this care, there exists an overarching problem of inadequate dedicated security controls to protect against network attacks, interference and potentially loss of life. The development of a tolerance level is essential and could serve as a catalyst to further evolve security measures for telehealth systems.

Questions for Discussion and Exploration

1. Identify 3 main ways that a small practice can protect telehealth data.

2. What are some other research studies that can be done that could lead to improvements in current policies?

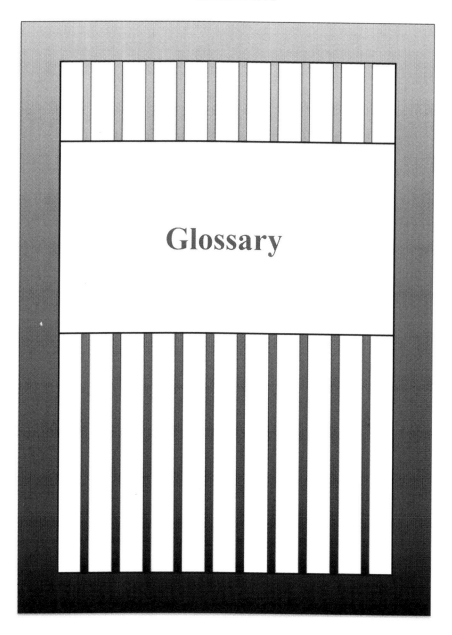

Glossary

Breach is defined as "the acquisition, access, use, or disclosure of protected health information in a manner which compromises the security or privacy of the protected health information" ("Breach Notification for Unsecured Protected Health Information", 2009, p. 42743).

Encryption is "the use of an algorithmic process to transform data into a form in which there is a low probability of assigning meaning without use of a confidential process or key" ("HIPAA Security Rule", 2007).

Health Insurance Portability and Accountability Act (HIPAA) is a federal Act instituted, in 1996, as a set of requirements for transmitting health data electronically. HIPAA supports greater accessibility to health data (especially in regard to insurance and research purposes) through electronic means, which also results in streamlined costs. Additionally, HIPAA was developed with the intent to aid in discovering fraud and negligent use of telehealth data. (Chaikind, Hearne, Lyke, Redhead, Stone, Franco, & Stevens, 2004).

HIPAA Breach Notification Rule is a law implemented in the HITECH Act that requires facilities that suffer a health information technology breach impacting 500 or more individuals to report the incident to the Department of Health and Human Services ("Breach Notification for Unsecured Protected Health Information", 2009).

HIPAA Security Rule "establishes national standards to protect individuals' electronic personal health information that is created, received, used, or maintained by a covered entity. The Security Rule requires appropriate administrative, physical and technical safeguards to ensure the confidentiality, integrity, and security of electronic protected health information" ("HIPAA Security Rule", 2007).

Health Information Technology (HIT) refers to the use of health-based technology infrastructures that allow for health data storage and collaboration components (Brailer & Thompson, 2004).

Health Information Technology for Economic and Clinical Health Act (HITECH) is an addendum to HIPAA that was instituted in 2009 by U.S. President Barack Obama. As a result of the Act, $22 billion dollars was allotted to improve policies and the utilization of health information technology (HIT). The HITECH addendum requires breaches to be reported to the HHS and also holds involved business associates accountable to regulations and to assume some responsibility in a related facilities security breaches to facilities. The security and privacy of data is an important component of this act (Klosek, 2010).

Interoperable Telesurgical Protocol (ITP) is a secure framework that is open for data transmissions between telesurgical robots and operators that is open for data transmissions between telesurgical robots and operators (Coble, Wang, Chu, & Li, 2010).

Security Controls are the physical, technical, and administrative security methods applied to a computer system (Northcutt, 2009).

Telehealth is health care that is administered via remote communications (Long & Long, 2002).

Telemedicine is the remote delivery of clinical medical services, using IT and electronic systems (American Telemedicine Association, 2006).

Telesurgery is surgery that is performed by a doctor that is in a different location than the patient, with the use of specialized surgical robot (Challacombe et al., 2006).

Telesurgical Robot System (TRS) is a system consisting of two major components, a "surgeon side" that receives direction from an operator in one location and a "patient side" that has surgical robotic arms and tools to perform an operation in another location. Zeus Systems and DaVinci Systems are TRSs (Marescaux et al., 2002).

Trauma Pod is a Pentagon-funded telesurgical operating room that can be assembled in locations without surgical facilities, particularly in war zones.

Tolerance level is defined as a set acceptable number of breaches that when exceeded, results in enforced consequences.

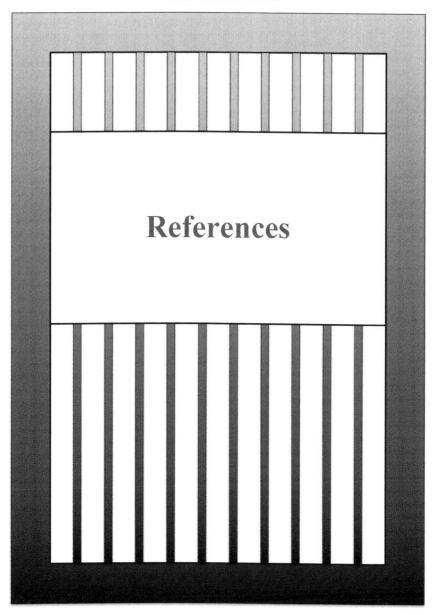

References

REFERENCES

American Telemedicine Association. (2006, May). *Telemedicine, telehealth, and health information technology: An ATA issue paper*. Retrieved from http://www.americantelemed.org/docs/default-source/policy/telemedicine-telehealth-and-health-information-technology.pdf?sfvrsn=8

Bhavani, Y., & Vijaya, Y. (2012). Background of surgical robos and robotics in different surgeries. *International Journal of Computer Science and Technology, 3*(1), 129-136. Retrieved from http://www.docstoc.com/Docs/Document-Detail-Google.aspx?doc_id=113046329#

Bonaci, T., & Chizeck, H.J. (2012, August). *Surgical telerobotics meets information security*. Paper presented at the Twenty First USENIX Security Symposium, Bellevue, WA. Retrieved from http://automation.berkeley.edu/RSS2012Workshop/abstract1.pdf

Brailer, D., & Thompson, T. (2004). *Health IT strategic framework*. Washington, DC: Department of Health and Human Services.

Breach Notification for Unsecured Protected Health Information, 74 Fed. Reg. 42,743 (2009) (to be codified at 45 C.F.R. pts 160 and 164).

Breen, G. M., & Matusitz, J. (2010). An evolutionary examination of telemedicine: A health and computer-mediated communication perspective. *Social Work in Public Health, 25*(1), 59-71.

Breen, G., Wan, T., & Ortiz, J. (2010). Information technology adoption in rural health clinics: A theoretical analysis. *Journal of Information Technology Impact, 10*(1), 1-14. Retrieved from http://www.jiti.net/v10/jiti.v10n1.001-014.pdf

Cason, J., & Brannon, J. (2011). Telehealth regulatory and legal considerations: Frequently asked questions. *International Journal of Telerehabilitation, 3*(2), 15-18. Retrieved from http://www.google.com/url?sa=t&rct=j&q=telehealth%20regulatory%20and%20legalconsiderations%3A%20frequently%20asked%20questions&source=web&cd=1&cad=rja&ved=0CCYQFjAA&url=http%3A%2F%2Ftelerehab.pitt.edu%2Fojs%2Findex.php%2FTelerehab%2Farticle%2Fdownload%2F6077%2F6339&ei=3_ILUMGMLOjj0QHnpoDgCg&usg=AFQjCNH1iTV1

hothaCPWgACBagY8nBnRZQ

Chaikind, H., Hearne, J., Lyke, B., Redhead, S., Stone, J., Franco, C., & Stevens, G. (2004). The Health Insurance Portability and Accountability ACT (HIPAA): Overview and analyses. Hauppauge, New York: Novinka Books.

Challacombe, B., Kavoussi, L., Patriciu, A., Stoianovici, D., & Dasgupta, P. (2006, November). Technology Insight: Telementoring and telesurgery in urology. *Natural Clinical Practice Urology, 3*(11). Retrieved from http://urobotics.urology.jhu.edu/pub/2006-challacombe-nature.pdf

Channel Insider (2011, August). Millions affected by health care data breaches since 2009. *Channel Insider.* Retrieved from http://www.channelinsider.com/c/a/Security/Millions-Affected-by-Health-Care-Data-Breaches-Since-2009-107573/

Charette, R. (2012, December 12). Cybercriminals hold Australian medical clinic electronic patient records hostage. *IEEE Spectrum: Inside Technology.* Retrieved from http://spectrum.ieee.org/riskfactor/telecom/security/cybercrimina ls-hold-australian-medical-clinic-electronic-patient-records-hostage

Chee, W.S.A. (2007). IT security in biomedical imaging informatics: The hidden vulnerability. *Journal of Mechanics in Medicine and Biology, 7*(1), 101-106.

Cisco. (2008). *Cisco adaptive wireless intrusion prevention system: Protecting information in motion.* Retrieved from Cisco website http://www.cisco.com/c/en/us/products/collateral/wireless/adapti ve-wireless-ips-software/solution_overview_c22-478925.pdf

Cisco. (2013). *Top children's hospital improves patient experience.* Retrieved from Cisco website http://www.cisco.com/en/US/prod/collateral/voicesw/ps6788/vca llcon/ps556/case_study_c36-726720.pdf

Claburn, T. (2009, May). Virginia Health Data Potentially Held Hostage. *InformationWeek: Dark Reading.* Retrieved from http://www.darkreading.com/attacks-and-breaches/virginia-health-data-potentially-held-hostage/d/d-id/1079193?

Coble, K., Wang, W., Chu, B., & Li, Z. (2010, November). Secure software attestation for military telesurgical robot systems. Paper presented at the 2010 Military Communications Conference - Unclassified Program - Cyber Security and Network Management, San Jose, CA. Retrieved from http://coitweb.uncc.edu/~wwang22/Research/papers/Milcom10-Wang.pdf

Cooper, T., & Collman, J. (2005). Managing information security and privacy in healthcare data mining: State of the art. In H.Chen, S.Fuller, C.Friedman, & W. Hersh (Eds.), *Medical informatics: Knowledge management and data mining in biomedicine* (pp. 97-137). New York, NY: Springer.

Costa, D. (2007, December 25). Your Body, Online. *PC Magazine*, pp. 60.

Craig, J., & Patterson, V. (2005). Introduction to the practice of telemedicine. *Journal of Telemedicine and Telecare*, 11, 3-9. Retrieved from http://telemedicina6.unifesp.br/set/curso/2006-06-19-pgsaude/Fundamental_IntroductiontothePracticeofTelemedicine.pdf

Creswell, J. W. (2004). *Educational research: Planning, conducting, and evaluating quantitative and qualitative research.* Upper Saddle River, NJ: Pearson.

Dagtas, S., Pekhteryev, G., Sahinoğlu, Z., Cam, H., & Challa, N. (2008). Real-time and secure wireless health monitoring. *International Journal of Telemedicine and Applications.*

Davidson, C.M., & Santorelli, M.J. (2009). *The impact of broadband on telemedicine.* Retrieved from the New York Law School, Advanced Communications Law & Policy Institute website: http://www.nyls.edu/user_files/1/3/4/30/83/BroadbandandTelemedicine.pdf

Deloitte. (2011). *Privacy and security in health care: A fresh look* (Issue Brief). Retrieved from http://www.deloitte.com/assets/Dcom-UnitedStates/Local%20Assets/Documents/Health%20Reform%20Issues%20Briefs/US_CHS_PrivacyandSecurityinHealthCare_022111.pdf

Desai, N., Krause, B., & Gemmill-Toyama, M. (2009). Health information technology in the United States: Can planning lead to reality?. *Eurohealth,15*(2), 26-28. Retrieved from

http://www2.lse.ac.uk/LSEHealthAndSocialCare/pdf/Desai%20v
15n2.pdf

Dimitropoulos, L.L. (2007). *Privacy and security solutions for interoperable health information exchange* (RTI Project No. 0209825.000.009). Retrieved from RTI International website: http://www.rti.org/pubs/fip_execsumm.pdf

Dimitropoulos, L., & Rizk, S. (2009). A state-based approach to privacy and security for interoperable health information exchange. *Health Affairs, 28*(2), 428-434. Retrieved from http://content.healthaffairs.org/content/28/2/428.full.pdf

District of Columbia Department of Health Care Finance. (n.d.). *FY2012-2014 strategic plan.* Retrieved from http://dhcf.dc.gov/sites/default/files/dc/sites/dhcf/publication/atta chments/DHCFStrategicPlanFY12-14.pdf

Eckhardt, J., Mühlbauer, T., AlTurki, M., Meseguer, J., & Wirsing, M. (2012). Stable availability under denial of service attacks through formal patterns. *Lecture Notes in Computer Science, 7212,* 78-93. Retrieved from http://link.springer.com/search?facet-author=%22Jonas+Eckhardt%22

Environmental Criteria and Standards, 24 C.F.R. § 51 *et seq.* (2007).

Fong, B., Fong, A.C.M, & Li, C.K. (2011). *Telemedicine technologies: Information technologies in medicine and telehealth.* United Kingdom: John Wiley & Sons, Ltd.

Garg, V. (2009). *Security concerns in telecare and telemedicine* (Master's Thesis). Retrieved from https://www.cerias.purdue.edu/assets/pdf/bibtex_archive/2009-11.pdf

Garg, V., & Brewer, J. (2011). Telemedicine security: A systematic review. *Journal of Diabetes Science and Technology, 5*(3), 768-777. Retrieved from http://www.ncbi.nlm.nih.gov/pmc/articles/PMC3192643/?tool=p ubmed

Geneiatakis, D., Dagiuklas, T., Kambourakis, G., Lambrinoudakis, C., Gritzalis, S., Ehlert, S., & Sisalem, D. (2006). Survey of security vulnerabilities in session initiation protocol. *IEEE Communication Surveys, 8*(3), 68-81. Retrieved from

http://mediatools.cs.ucl.ac.uk/nets/dos/export/1439/sip/reference/
papers/IEEE_COMSURVEYS_dagiuklas.pdf

Gravetter, F. J., & Forzano, L. B. (2011). *Research methods for the
behavioral sciences.* Belmont, California: Cengage Learning.

Hanley, E.J., & Broderick, T. J. (2005). Telerobotic surgery. *Operative
Techniques in General Surgery, 7*(4), 170-181. Retrieved from
http://www.christiansurgeon._com/
Telerobotic%20surgery%20Op%20Tech
%20Gen%20Surg%202005.pdf

Health Insurance Reform: Security Standards; Final Rule, 68 Fed. Reg.
34 (2003) (to be codified at 45 C.F.R. pts 160, 162, and 164).

Health Information Technology for Economic and Clinical Health
(HITECH) Act, Title XIII of Division A and Title IV of Division
B of the American Recovery and Reinvestment Act of 2009
(ARRA), Pub. L. No. 111-5 (Feb. 17, 2009), *codified at* 42
U.S.C. §§300jj *et seq.*; §§17901 *et seq.*

Healthcare IT News Staff. (2012, October 29). Verizon releases industry-
by-industry snapshots of cybercrime, based on the data breach
investigations report series. *Healthcare IT News.* Retrieved from
http://www.healthcareitnews.com/press-release/verizon-releases-
industry-industry-snapshots-cybercrime-based-data-breach-
investigatio

Heiman, G. (2011). *Behavioral sciences STAT.* Belmont, California:
Cengage Learning.

Hein, M. (2009). Telemedicine: An important force in the transformation
of healthcare. Retrieved from
http://ita.doc.gov/td/health/telemedicine_2009.pdf

HIPAA Security Rule, 45 C.F.R. § 160 *et seq.* (2007).

HIPAA Security Rule, 45 C.F.R. § 162 *et seq.* (2007).

HIPAA Security Rule, 45 C.F.R. § 164 *et seq.* (2007).

Horowitz, B. (2011, November). Cisco boosts mobility, security for
HealthPresence telehealth platform. *Eweek.* Retrieved from
http://www.eweek.com/c/a/Health-Care-IT/Cisco-Boosts-
Mobility-Security-for-HealthPresence-Telehealth-Platform-
769645/

Horton, K. (2008). The use of telecare for people with chronic
obstructive

Istepanian R. S. H., & Lacal, J.C. (2003). Emerging mobile communication technologies for health: Some imperative notes on m-health. *Proceedings of the Twenty-Fifth International Conference of the IEEE Engineering in Medicine and Biology Society, 2*, 1414-1416.

Jointer, S. (2011). *Lattices of expert systems and their application in the telehealth domain* (Doctoral Dissertation). Retrieved from http://proquest.umi.com/pqdweb?did=2337201901&sid=8& Fmt=2&clientId=62408&RQT=309&VName=PQD

Joint Task Force Transformation Initiative. (2009). Recommended Security Controls for Federal Information Systems and Organizations (NIST Special Publication 800-53, Revision 3). Gaithersburg, MD: National Institute of Standards and Technology. Retrieved from http://csrc.nist.gov/publications/nistpubs/800-53-Rev3/sp800-53-rev3-final_updated-errata_05-01-2010.pdf

Kramer, D.B., Baker, M., Ransford, B., Molina-Markham, A., Stewart, Q., Fu, K., & Reynolds, M. (2012). Security and privacy qualities of medical devices: An analysis of FDA postmarket surveillance. *PLoS ONE, 7*(7), e40200. Retrieved from http://www.plosone.org/article/info%3Adoi%2F10.1371%2Fjour nal.pone.0040200

Lee, G., & Thuraisingham, B. (2012). Cyberphysical systems security applied to telesurgical robotics. *Computer Standards & Interfaces, 34*, 225–229. Retrieved from http://www.utdallas.edu/~bxt043000/Publications/Journal-Papers/DAS/J67_Cyberphysical%20Systems%20Security%20A pplied%20to%20Telesurgical%20Robotics.pdf

Liu, Q. (2008). *Securing telehealth applications in a web-based e-health portal.* Retrieved from http://proquest.umi.com.login.capitol-college.edu:2048/pqdweb? index=36&did=1574047031&SrchMode=1&sid=8&Fmt=2&VI nst=PROD&VType=PQD&RQT=309&VName=PQD&TS=132 3749046&clientId=62408

Luxton, D.D., Kayl, R.A., & Mishkind, M.C. (2012). mHealth data security: The need for HIPAA-compliant standardization. *Telemedicine Journal and E-Health: The Official Journal of the*

American Telemedicine Association, 18(4), 284-288. doi: 10.1089/tmj.2011.0180.

Lyons, P., & Doueck, H. (2010). *The Dissertation: From beginning to end.* New York, New York: Oxford University Press.

Maji, A. K., Mukhoty, A., Majumdar, A. K., Mukhopadhyay, J., Sural, S., Paul, S. & Majumdar, B. (2008, January). *Security analysis and implementation of web-based telemedicine services with a four-tier architecture.* Paper presented at the First International ICST Workshop on Connectivity, Mobility and Patients' Comfort, Tampere, Finland. Abstract retrieved from http://eudl.eu/article.php?id=2518

Marescaux, J., Leroy, J., Rubino, F., Smith, M., Vix, M., Simone, M., & Mutter, D. (2002). Transcontinental robot-assisted remote telesurgery: Feasibility and potential applications. *Annals of Surgery, 253*(4). Retrieved from http://www.ncbi.nlm.nih.gov/pmc/articles/PMC1422462/

Maryland Health Care Commission. (n.d.). *Health information technology state plan: FY 2011-FY2014.* Retrieved from http://mhcc.dhmh.maryland.gov/hit/hiePolicyBoard/Documents/ mhcc.maryland.gov/hit_state_plan_fy2011_2014_final_web_rep ortsection.pdf %20HIE%20Strategic%20and%20Operational%20Plan.pdf

Matusitz, J., & Breen, G. (2007). Telemedicine: Its effects on health communication. *Health Communication, 21*(1), 73–83. Retrieved from http://www.uapd.com/wp-content/uploads/Telemedicine-Its-Effects-on-Health-Communication.pdf

Nagy, B. (2006, September). Telemedicine's depth now going beyond rural areas: Advancing technology brings care to patients in more places through real-time interaction or store-and-forward processes. *Managed Healthcare Executive.* Retrieved from http://managedhealthcareexecutive.modernmedicine.com/mhe/ar ticle/articleDetail.jsp?id=368114

Navas, K.A., Thampy, S.A., & Sasikumar, M. (2007). EPR hiding in medical images for telemedicine. *International Journal of Biological and Medical Sciences, 3*(1), 44-47. Retrieved from http://www.waset.org/journals/ijbls/v3/v3-1-6.pdf.

Nebraska Information Technology Commission (2012). *Nebraska operational*

Office for the Advancement for Telehealth Health Resources and Services Administration, Department of Health and Human Services (2003). *Telemedicine licensure report.* Retrieved from http://www.hrsa.gov/ruralhealth/about/ telehealth/licenserpt03.pdf

Office of the National Coordinator for Health Information Technology. (2009). State health information exchange cooperative agreement program. Retrieved from https://www.grantsolutions.gov/gs/preaward/previewPublicAnno uncement.do?id=10534

Ponemon Institute. (2014). *Fourth annual benchmark study on patient privacy & data security.* Retrieved from http://lpa.idexpertscorp.com/acton/attachment/6200/f-012c/1/-/-/-/-/ID%20Experts%204th%20Annual%20Patient%20Privacy%20 %26%20Data%20Security%20Report%20FINAL%20%281%29 .pdf

Rosen, J., & Hannaford, B. (2006, October). Doc at a Distance: Robot surgeons promise to save lives in remote communities, war zones, and disaster-stricken areas. *IEEE Spectrum: Inside Technology.* Retrieved from http://spectrum.ieee.org/biomedical /devices/doc-at-a-distance/0

RSA. (2012). *Cybercrime and the healthcare industry.* Retrieved from RSA website: http://www.rsa.com/products/consumer/whitepapers/11030_CY

Schumacher, R.M., Patterson, E.S., North, R., Zhang, J., Lowry, S.Z., Quinn, M.T., & Ramaiah, M. (2011). NIST draft guidance on technical evaluation, testing, and validation of the usability of electronic health records. Retrieved from http://www.nist.gov/healthcare/usability/upload/Draft_EUP_09_ 28_11.pdf

Shimizu, S., Nakashima, N., Okamura, K., Han, H., & Tanaka, M. (2007, October). Telesurgery system with original-quality moving images over high-speed internet: Expansion within the Asia-Pacific region. *Journal of Laparoendoscopic & Advanced Surgical Techniques, 17* (3). Retrieved from

http://content.ebscohost.com/pdf19_22/pdf/
2007/4C5/01Oct07/26863235.pdf
?T=P&P=AN&K=26863235&S=R&D=aph&EbscoContent=dG
JyMMvl7ESep7A4wtvhOLCmr0meqK5Ss6e4Ta%2BWxWXS
&ContentCustomer=dGJyMPGpsEiwrLNKuePfgeyx44Dt6flA

Siau, K., & Shen, Z. (2006, June). Mobile healthcare informatics.
Medical Informatics and the Internet in Medicine, 31(2), 89-99.
Retrieved from http://content.
ebscohost.com/pdf18_21/pdf/2006/BAX/01Jun06/21193840.pdf
?T=P&P=AN&K=21193840&S=R&D=aph&EbscoContent=dG
JyMMvl7ESep7A4wtvhOLCmr0meqK9Sr6m4TbGWxWXS&C
ontentCustomer=dGJyMPGpsEiwrLNKuePfgeyx44Dt6flA

Spivack, R. (2005). Innovation in telehealth and a role for the
government. *Studies in Health Technology and Informatics, 118,*
32-42. Retrieved from
http://www.atp.nist.gov/eao/innov_telehealth_role_gov_2004.pd
f

Tozal, M.E., Wang, Y., Al-Shaer, E., Sarac, K., Thuraisingham, B., &
Chu, B. (2011). Adaptive information coding for secure and
reliable wireless telesurgery communications. *Mobile Networks
and Applications,* 1-15. doi:10.1007/s11036-011-0333-3

Ungerleider, N. (2012, August 15). Medical cybercrime: The next
frontier. *Fast Company.* Retrieved from
http://www.fastcompany.com/3000470/medical-cybercrime-
next-frontier

U.S. Department of Health & Human Services. (n.d.). *Audit program
protocol.* Retrieved from
http://www.hhs.gov/ocr/privacy/hipaa/enforcement/audit/protoco
l.html

U.S. Department of Health & Human Services. (2011). Annual update of
the HHS poverty guidelines. *Federal register: The daily journal
of the United States government.* Retrieved from
https://www.federalregister.gov/articles/2011/01/20/2011-
1237/annual-update-of-the-hhs-poverty-

U.S. Department of Health & Human Services. (2013a). *Breaches
affecting 500 or more individuals.* Retrieved from
http://www.hhs.gov/ocr/privacy/hipaa/administrative/breachnotif

icationrule/breachtool.html

U.S. Department of Health & Human Services. (2013b). *How OCR enforces the HIPAA privacy & security rules*. Retrieved from http://www.hhs.gov/ocr/privacy/hipaa/enforcement/process/how ocrenforces.html

U.S. Department of Health & Human Services. (2013c). *What OCR considers during intake & review*. Retrieved from http://www.hhs.gov/ocr/privacy/hipaa/enforcement/process/what ocrconsiders.html

Verizon. (2012). *DBIR industry snapshot: Healthcare*. Retrieved from http://www.verizonenterprise.com/resources/reports/rp_dbir-industry-snapshot-healthcare_en_xg.pdf

von Urff, C. (2004). *Facilitating delivery of advanced telemedicine services to rural areas and lesser developed countries through a new hybrid telecommunications system with prescribed end-to-end performance criteria* (Doctoral Dissertation, Capella University). Retrieved from http://proquest.umi.com/pqdlink?did=1404355171&Fmt=6&clientId=62408&RQT=309&VName=PQD

Watzlaf, V., Fahima, R., Moeini, S., & Firouzan, P. (2010). VoIP for telerehabilitation: A risk analysis for privacy, security, and HIPAA compliance. *International Journal of Telerehabilitation, 2*(2), 3-14. doi:10.5195/IJT.2010.6056

Watzlaf, V., Fahima, R., Moeini, S., Matusow, L. & Firouzan, P. (2011). VoIP for telerehabilitation: A risk analysis for privacy, security, and HIPAA compliance –part II. *International Journal of Telerehabilitation, 3*(1), 3-10. doi: 10.5195/IJT.2011.6070

White, P. (2002). Legal issues in teleradiology—distant thoughts!. *The British Institute of Radiology, 75*, 201-206. Retrieved from http://bjr.birjournals.org/cgi/reprint/ 75/891/201

Wozak, F., Schabetsberger, T., & Ammmenwerth, E (2007). End-to-end security in telemedical networks – A practical guideline. *International Journal of Medical Informatics, 76*, 484-490. Retrieved from http://iig.umit.at/dokumente/z44.pdf

Xiao, Y., Shen, X., Sun, B., & Cai, L. (2006, April). Security and privacy in RFID and applications in telemedicine. *IEEE Communications*

Magazine, 64-72. Retrieved from http://bbcr.uwaterloo.ca/ ~xshen/paper/2006/sapira.pdf

Zain, J., & Clarke, M. (2005, March). *Security in telemedicine: Issues in watermarking medical images*. Paper presented at the Third International Conference: Sciences of Electronic, Technologies of Information and Telecommunications, Tunisia. Retrieved from http://www.setit.rnu.tn/last_edition/setit2005/applications/366.pd f

Zawada, E., Herr, P., Larson, D., Fromm, R., Kapaska, D., & Erikson, D. (2009). Impact of an intensive care unit telemedicine program on a rural health care system. Postgraduate Medicine, *121*(3), 159-170. Retrieved from http://www.americantelemed.org/files/public/membergroups/tele icu/Impact%20of%20an%20Intensive%20Care%20Unit%20Tele medicine%20Program%20on%20a%20Rural%20Health%20Car e%20System.pdf

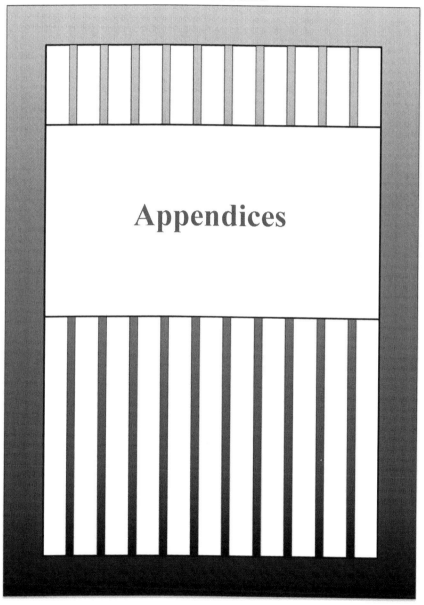

Appendices

APPENDIX A: INSTRUMENTATION

1. What are the total percentages of telehealth breaches per medium type for the United States?

2. What are the total percentages of telehealth breaches per breach type for the United States?

3. What are the most prevalent mediums involved in U.S. telehealth breaches?

4. What are the most prevalent telehealth breach types occurring in the United States?

5. What was the total number of U.S. telehealth breaches per semi-annual interval?

APPENDIX B: SUMMARY OF STUDY RESULTS

At the time of data retrieval breach counts that classified as telehealth breaches (as defined in this study) were as follows:

Telehealth breach counts from 2009-2012 in semi-annual increments

Time	Breach Counts	Variance
2009-2nd half	33	start
2010-1st half	79	increase
2010-2nd half	72	decrease
2011-1st half	49	decrease
2011-2nd half	64	increase
2012-1st half	76	increase
2012-2nd half	74	decrease

Note: *A breach may have occurred over multiple semi-annual increments

- Telehealth could:

  - Improve efficiency & collaboration

  - Decrease health care costs by $500 billion dollars over 15 years (Costa, 2007)

- Encryption should be used as a security mechanism

  - Supported by NIST Special Publications

- States may vary in their requirements for facility security plans

  - Plans are required for funding by HITECH

- No telehealth breach tolerance levels exist

APPENDIX C: TELEHEALTH AFFILIATES FEEDBACK QUESTIONS

1. What state is your telehealth facility or telehealth program located in?

2. Are you a medical physician, an affiliate of a telehealth program (i.e. a director, consultant, etc.), or both?

3. What type of media is most commonly used in your practice (or programs you are affiliated with) [multiple selections are allowed]?

4. Even though HIPAA imposes fines and criminal punishment on facilities for telehealth breaches, there is currently no breach threshold. While there may not be a legislated threshold, what does your practice or program use in order to quantify what is an acceptable breach count?

5. Has your practice or program used a threshold from another industry as a benchmark for breach acceptability (i.e. the insurance industry)?

6. What are your opinions on a facility being required to submit and carry out a plan of action after a threshold of breaches, each affecting 500 or more individuals, occurs within a 6-month time period?

APPENDIX D: SECURITY & POLICY IMPROVEMENT RECOMMENDATIONS

I.   HIPAA should employ a breach threshold standard

II.   Data Encryption should be required for all telehealth systems that hold PII, and not just noted as "addressable"

III.   A deeper correlation needs to be made in regard to HHS documented breaches and possible improvements for HIPAA

IV.   Breach-reporting data needs to be more detailed (categorizing breach types or mediums as "others" introduce limitations in research efforts)

V.   Organizations need to implement enforced physical security measures

VI.   Consolidated Commercial Security tools should be used:
   i.   Intrusion Prevention Systems (IPS)
   ii.   Unified Threat Management Systems (UTM)

APPENDIX E: NEWSWORTHY INCIDENTS

- Veteran Affairs Incidents
  - May 2006: Laptop stolen from analyst's home; affected 26.5 million (name, DOB, SSN)

- Virginia's Prescription Monitoring Program
  - April 2009: Hacked into web site; affected 8 million; requested $10 million ransom
  - VA Prescription Monitoring Program Hacker's Note: *"Attention Virginia! I have your [expletive]! In *my* possession, right now, are 8,257,378 patient records and a total of 35,548,087 prescriptions. Also, I made an encrypted backup and deleted the original. Unfortunately for Virginia, their backups seem to have gone missing, too. Uh oh :(For $10 million, I will gladly send along the password."* (Claburn, 2009)

- Southerland HealthCare Solutions
  - April 2014: 8 computers stolen during break in; affected 338,700 (name, DOB, SSN, address, medical information)

APPENDIX F: ALL QUESTIONS FOR DISCUSSION & EXPLORATION

1. Identify and discuss 3 telehealth cybercrime incidents in the last year. How could they have possibly been prevented?

2. Identify a U.S. state's telehealth strategic or operational plan. Identify how it could be improved.

3. Discuss whether encryption for telehealth should be required or whether it should remain as addressable.

4. List and explain at least 3 major issues that can result from a hacked telesurgery.

5. Explain the pros and cons of the following solutions being developed: images, smart cards, RSA tokens, SSR-UDP, Secure ITP, and RFID.

6. List and discuss 3 suggestions from NIST standards that can help protect telehealth systems.

7. Research and discuss DARPA and other government telehealth initiatives to help save individuals in war zones.

8. Research the telemedicine/telehealth black market and identify reasons for why hacking and IT incidents are the most common types of breaches.

9. Identify 2 EMR platforms. Discuss the differences and similarities in the 2 platforms' security components.

10. List and explain how a breach threshold could positively impact a reduction in telehealth breaches.

11. Explain why you think an explicit breach threshold has not yet been clearly outlined as a regulation.

12. Identify 3 main ways that a small practice can protect telehealth data.

13. What are some other research studies that can be done that could lead to improvements in current policies?

APPENDIX G: POLICIES & DOCUMENTATION TO EXPLORE

- Health Information Portability and Accountability Act (HIPAA)

- Health Information Technology for Economic and Clinical Health (HITECH) Act
  - o Breach Notification Rule
  - o Security Rule

- American Recovery and Reinvestment Act (ARRA)

- Federal Information Security Management Act (FISMA)

- NIST SPECIAL PUBLICATION 800-66 REVISION 1 Guidance for HIPAA Required Access Control and Transmission Security

- NIST SPECIAL PUBLICATION 800-53 REVISION 3 Guidance on Access Enforcement

- NISTIR 7497 Guidance on Encryption

- How the Office for Civil Rights (OCR) Enforces HIPAA Privacy & Security Rules

- HIPAA Civil Penalties Imposed by 42 USC § 1320d-5 and ARRA

- HIPAA Criminal Penalties Imposed by 42 USC § 1320d-5 and ARRA

APPENDIX H: RESEARCH AREAS FOR COURSES

- **Future Research Recommendation #1:**

  Research the potential correlations between implemented security mechanisms and breach rates, in efforts to establish a threshold

- **Future Research Recommendation #2:**

  Examine the possible relationship between telehealth security documentation and the breach levels of small telehealth facilities

CONTACT THE AUTHOR

Contact Dr. Seria D. Lakes at **Dr.SeriaLakes@gmail.com** for speaking engagements, discounts on bulk book purchases, and questions.

90422935R00075

Made in the USA
Middletown, DE
23 September 2018